Handling Dengue Fever:

The Complete Information on Surviving the Disease

Written by

Judy Medina

Copyright © by Dr. Judy M. Medina 2023. All rights reserved.

Any copying or other form of duplication of this work must get the publisher's permission. This prevents the data within from being electronically transmitted, kept in a database, or both.

Without the author's consent, the document may not be copied, scanned, faxed, or retained in whole or in part.

Table of Contents

Introduction

Global medical services are put to the test by the virus responsible for dengue fever, a tenacious and powerful foe that stalks equatorial environments, inflicting its mark on populations.

Dengue fever is a virus that should be taken seriously as it is spread via the sly bite of Aedes mosquitoes, which are capable of making people susceptible to its wide-ranging and frequently unforeseen symptoms. Dengue fever brings a complicated story that includes not just the biological components of the infectious agent but also the societal, economic, and environmental elements that facilitate its propagation, ranging from the fevered heat of scorching temperatures as well as the Joint-wrenching discomfort that frequently follows its emergence.

By preventing mosquito bites, particularly during the daylight hours, you can reduce your risk of contracting dengue. Since there currently exists no specific treatment for dengue, it is managed using pain medications.

Causes of Dengue Fever

Dengue disease is brought on by one of the four dengue viruses. The dengue virus may get into the bloodstream and multiply when a mosquito biting you transmits the disease. You may feel ill due to the viral infection and your immune system's reaction.

The virus can damage blood components that help you create clots and give your blood vessels shape. Bleeding inside may result from this, combined with specific immune system-produced substances, causing blood to flow out of your vessels. This results in intense dengue symptoms, which can be fatal.

Storage of water and inadequate sanitation are further variables that contribute to its proliferation. Aedes mosquitoes can spawn in places with water-holding containers, including homes and public areas. Water containers that enable the reproduction of mosquitoes might build up as a result of poor sanitation and insufficient garbage removal.

Insufficient vector management can result in greater numbers of mosquitoes and increased rates of spread. Poor vector control procedures includes not sprinkling larvicide, and eliminating sources.

Climate circumstances:The breeding and activity of Aedes mosquitoes are supported by favorable climatic circumstances, which include scorching temperatures and humidity. The geographic distribution of these insects may be impacted by changes in climate, increasing the areas subject to risk for spread of dengue.

Poor Immunity: Following infection, people may develop resistance against a particular serotype of dengue in areas where the disease is prevalent. However, a condition known as enhancement of antibodies (EOA) can make dengue more severe following additional infections involving various serotypes.

Stages of Dengue Fever Attack

After a usual duration of gestation of about 5-7 days, dengue starts quickly and progresses through three stages: shivering, critical, and recovering stages.

In the phase of shivering;

■ Fever may be in dual-phase and persist for a period of 48 to 168 hours on average.

■ In addition, there may be additional indicators such as strong migraines, retro-orbital eye discomfort, joint, muscle, and pain in the bones.

■ Within the initial 1-2 days following commencement,

certain individuals experience facial redness and infused throat.

During the late shivering phase, around the point of temperature drop, warning indications of severe dengue include prolonged nausea, breathing problems, excruciating stomach pain, fluid buildup, mucosal bleeding, low blood pressure, and restlessness.

Critical Phase

Dengue's critical phase, which normally lasts 1 to 2 days, starts with abatement. The majority of sufferers see clinical improvement during this stage, but those who have significant vascular permeability may experience acute dengue within a few hours due to a significant rise in plasma leakage.

▪ Hemodilution, ascites, hypoalbuminemia, and effusions of the pleural cavity are possible symptoms for individuals with significant plasma leakage.

▪ As diastole blood pressure rises, physiological compensating systems initially preserve sufficient blood flow, that reduces the pressure of the pulse.

▪ Patients, particularly those who have been in chronic bleeding, can also experience serious hemorrhagic symptoms such as bloody stools and vomiting of blood.

■   Individuals might seem to be in good health despite first shock symptoms. However, if low blood pressure sets in, the systolic blood pressure quickly drops, and even with Corrected Platelet Recovery (CPR), irreversible shock and death may occur.

The patient approaches the convalescent phase when capillary leakage slows down and starts to take in leaked intravenous liquids as well as pleural fluid accumulation. An individual's hemodynamic condition becomes stable as their health increases, and urination follows. Due to the dilutional impact of the retained fluid, the patient's hemoglobin level becomes stable or may even decrease, and the white cell count typically starts to climb. Next, the number of platelets in the patient recovers.

■ The rash during the recovery phase may exfoliate and be itchy.

Thrombocytopenia, neutropenia, water intoxication, increased aspartate transaminase and alanine transaminase (ALT), and a normal red blood cell sedimentation rate are typical laboratory results.

How to detect if you have the Dengue Fever

Dengue fever frequently begins with minor symptoms that are similar to the flu, but it can eventually escalate to serious and perhaps fatal diseases.

Look out for the signs and symptoms that follow in both adults and children to see if you're suffering from dengue fever.

Adult Signs

The vast majority of dengue patients have little to no symptoms and recover in one to two weeks. Rarely, dengue can be fatal due to its severity.

When they do, symptoms often appear 4 –10 days after infection and continue for 2–7 days. Some signs could be:

- Rash
- An excruciating headache
- Aches in the muscles and joints
- Nausea
- Discomfort around the eyes
- High temperature (40°C)
- Vomiting and glandular enlargement.

Severe dengue is more likely to affect people who have already been infected once.

Strong dengue symptoms frequently appear after the illness has subsided. They include:

- Quick respiration
- Weariness
- Excruciating stomach discomfort
- Nasal bleeding
- Ongoing vomiting
- Anxiousness

Insist on immediate medical attention if you experience these serious symptoms.

Infants' Symptoms

Infants may have trouble distinguishing dengue symptoms from those of other common childhood diseases. If your kid gets a fever and exhibits any of the following signs, visit a doctor right away.

- Bruising and bleeding unusually via the nose and gums.
- Fever or low body temperature (96.8°F)
- Vomiting
- Tiredness, or inactivity.
- Rash

Preventing the Disease

Dengue disease prevention involves a mix of individual behaviors, group initiatives, and precautionary measures.

Here are a few methods to fend off dengue:

- **Spray insecticides**: Insecticides with N,N-Diethyl-meta-toluamide, picaridin, or other suggested components to expose skin and clothes, particularly during the early hours of the morning and late afternoon when the activity of mosquitoes is at its greatest.

- **Keep Your Environment Clean**: Get rid of rubbish and unwanted things that can gather water and serve as places for mosquitoes to breed properly. To avoid water buildup, keep your downspouts, pipes, and waterways clean.
- **Remove reproduction locations**: In stagnant water, Aedes mosquitoes can reproduce. Canisters that store water, including flower pots, buckets, used tires, and reservoir containers as well, should be routinely emptied, covered, or treated.

- **Employ Bed Nets**: If you live in a region with a significant dengue transmission rate, consider sleeping inside a bed net. Pick insecticide-treated nets if at all possible.

- **Use Protective Outfits**: To minimize skin contact, use lengthy-sleeved shirts, long trousers, gloves, and socks while in locations that have significant mosquito activity.

- **Installing Screen Windows and Doors**: To prevent mosquitoes in residential spaces, utilize window and door screens. Restore any broken screens to keep mosquitoes out.

- **Encourage Neighborhood Cleanups**: Organize neighborhood cleanup efforts to eliminate possible places for mosquito breeding. Invite your neighbors to contribute to the effort to reduce mosquito habitats.
- **Get Informed**: Use authoritative sources and health department advisories to keep up with local dengue epidemics, preventive measures, and control of mosquitoes initiatives.

- **Vaccination**: If an appropriate vaccine is authorized and readily available, consider getting immunized against dengue in accordance with the options and suggestions provided in your area.

- **Participate in Health Schemes**: Participate in local health officials' efforts to control mosquitoes, including larval control, and mosquito net distribution.

- **Travel Safety Measures**: Use insect repellents, put on protective clothing, and stay in lodgings with mosquito nets or shields if you're going to a place where dengue is prevalent.

- **Help Others Learn**: Promote preventing the spread of dengue in your neighborhood. Disseminate knowledge about how to get rid of mosquito breeding places and avoid getting bitten.

Herbal Remedy that works for Dengue Fever

These are some efficient natural treatments that can aid in reducing dengue symptoms. These treatments can lower your persistent fever and relieve some of the symptoms you are experiencing.

Here are several treatments that can help you manage dengue and its side effects.

▪ Papaya Juice

Papaya juice made from leaves is a fantastic treatment to boost the number of platelets as it decreases in dengue patients. Additionally, the juice made from papaya leaves boosts immunity, which aids in the treatment of dengue. Take some papaya leaves and smash them to release the juice in order to treat dengue with them. For best outcomes, you can drink just a little of papaya leaf juice twice every day.

▪ Pure Guava Juice

Guava juice contains a variety of nutrients. It contains a lot of vitamin C, a compound that boosts body defense. You can treat dengue fever by including fresh guava fruit juice in your diet. You are also going to receive additional health benefits from guava juice. Twice a day, sip a single glass of guava juice. In addition to juice, guava can also be eaten freshly.

- **Giloy Juice**

A recognized treatment for dengue fever is giloy juice. Giloy juice boosts body defense and metabolic processes. Effective defense against dengue fever is aided by a high degree of immunity. The patient feels better and the amount of platelets rises as a result.

Two little Giloy plant stems can be boiled in a glass of water. When the water is just a little warm, drink it. You can also make a cup of hot water with just a few drops of Giloy juice and sip it twice daily. However, be careful not to take too much of it.

- **Fenugreek Seeds**

Numerous nutrients included in fenugreek seeds aid in combating dengue fever. You could soak the seeds of fenugreek in a glass of hot water. Consume the water twice daily after letting it cool. Your health will gain additional advantages from fenugreek water's high fiber, vitamin K content, and vitamin C. Fenugreek drink will lower fever and strengthen your immune system.

Other food that improves immunity;

You can avoid getting dengue and may recover from dengue fever more quickly with an effective immune system. Robust immunity will additionally alleviate dengue's initial signs. You must include foods that improve immunity in your diet, such as citrus fruits, garlic, turmeric, almonds, bell peppers, and broccoli.

Diagnosis and Medical Treatment for Dengue Disease

Blood tests are used to diagnose dengue disease. In order to check for dengue virus, the doctor treating you will draw blood from you and then take it to a lab for analysis. Additionally, this could tell you whichever versions you have. Your doctor may order an examination of your blood to look for other infections that produce similar symptoms.

Dengue infection cannot be treated with a specific medication. Use acetaminophen-containing painkillers and stay away from aspirin-containing medications if you suspect you have dengue fever since they could worsen bleeding. Additionally, you ought to get enough of rest, hydration, and medical attention. In the first 24 hours after your fever has subsided, if your symptoms worsen, you should visit a hospital right once to be evaluated for problems.

Managing Food Irritability during Recovery

Food-related allergies are uncommonly brought on by dengue, but the healing cycle from a viral infection like the disease can occasionally leave patients with sensitive stomachs or compromised digestive systems.

Here are some broad guidelines for controlling food irritation during the healing process.

- **Beginning with mild foods**: Start with moderate, readily absorbed foods. Stick to simple soups, plain rice, bananas, plain toast, applesauce, and yogurt. These nourishing foods can aid with your appetite recovery and are easy on the stomach.

- **Hydration**: Water intake should be enough prior to and following dengue fever. For the benefit of the functioning of your digestive system and in helping to restore equilibrium of electrolytes. Consume enough water, clear liquids, and oral rehydration treatments.

- **Steer clear of spicy and oily foods**: This is because they can be difficult to digest and may aggravate your stomach. Once your digestive system is fully restored, stay away from these.

- **Regular Meals**: Eat smaller, more regular meals throughout the day rather than three large ones. This may make digestion simpler and help keep your stomach from being overloaded.

- **Minimize dairy products**: This is due to the fact that they can occasionally be difficult to digest, particularly if you have a sensitive stomach. Choose lactose-free alternatives, or consume plain yogurt in moderation as it provides probiotics that can help with digestion.

- **Consume fiber-rich foods**: Foods such as veggies, fruits, and whole grains. Fiber can help with digestion and control bowel motions, which may become uncontrollable during recovery.

Include lean proteins such as fish, bean curd, and lentils in your diet. When opposed to meats that are fatty, these are simpler to digest.

- **Ginger and peppermint**: Both of these ingredients are widely recognized for their calming effects on the stomach. To ease any discomfort, you might drink peppermint or tea made with ginger.

- **Probiotics**: Consuming dietary supplements or foods high in probiotics may assist with metabolism and the balance of beneficial intestinal bacteria return to normal. Some examples are sauerkraut, kimchi, kefir, and yogurt.

- **Chew Thoroughly**: Enjoy your meal and chew it completely. This can facilitate digesting and ease stomach stress.

- **Ignore Trigger Foods**: If you discover that something you're eating is making you uncomfortable or agitated, avoid it until your stomach is feeling better.

A good meal would be light congee. The same might be said about noodles cooked in clear soup.

Give your body the time it needs to fully recuperate by taking it easy and being patient. Don't jump right back onto your usual diet. Pay attention to your state of health and change your diet as necessary.

The After Effect

After an illness, pregnancy, emotionally trying circumstances, etc., the body enters an unusual state. This triggers the body to stop the hair's growth cycle, resulting in strands of hair falling out.

The term for it is TELOGEN EFFLUVIUM. In 90% of cases, it comes right back by itself after a few months, but in the other ten percent, the growth that follows is poor.

Patients should see a medical professional for additional assistance because such cases require external as well as internal treatment to promote hair growth.

Other effects could be reduction in blood platelets.

Vitamin A, which is found in spinach and is essential for keeping healthy skin and mucous membranes, may be helpful when recovering from dengue and healthy platelets.

It's important to remember that while nutrients are beneficial for overall health, there isn't a single food that is capable of increasing the number of platelets in dengue infections. Managing dengue fever requires medical attention and surveillance since platelet counts might decline considerably during the illness. It's crucial to heed medical guidance and therapy recommendations from healthcare professionals.

Conclusion

Tropical and subtropical regions are affected by the viral disease dengue fever, which is spread by mosquitoes.

A second infection with the virus increases the risk of having a serious illness. There are four different strains of the virus that causes dengue fever, and it appears that tolerance to one strain makes infection by another strain more deadly.

After a usual incubation period of five to seven days, dengue starts quickly and progresses through three stages: shivering, critical, and convalescent. The infection is typically more severe the second time that a person contracts dengue than the first. Once exposed to a single strain, a person's body develops resistance against that particular virus strain.

Each subsequent reinfection is far riskier than the one before it. Pain is reduced with analgesics like acetaminophen (paracetamol). To relieve the dehydration brought on by diarrhea, it's imperative to drink a lot of water. Without therapy, the problem often gets better with time. An infectious disease specialist, however, can handle tropical infectious disorders. You should visit the emergency room of your neighborhood hospital if you get sick again.

www.ingramcontent.com/pod-product-compliance
Lightning Source LLC
Chambersburg PA
CBHW070749260726
48660CB00007B/3026